Honey & I:
101 Thoughts, One Thought a Day
In Celebration of Honey and Bees

All Copyright 2011.

Note to the Reader

Honey & I

~101 Thoughts, One Thought a Day~
In Celebration of Honey and Bees

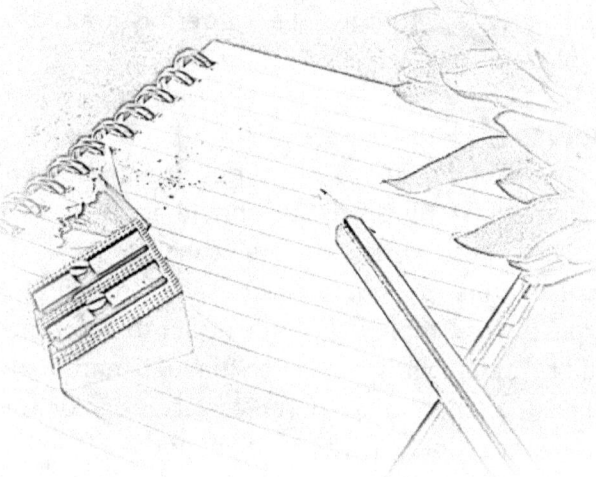

Preface

I hardly see the bees here. But I eat much of their food (sometimes too much) and have benefitted much from it. And I spend much time (way too much at times) reading, thinking, and writing about honey and the bees. What I have placed on the pages of this book speaks of my frenzy love for honey, my high regard for its intelligence as a healthful food, my utter amazement at its goodness to our body, my chagrin when honey critics attempt to smother my beliefs, my deep admiration of the lively sparks, the flowering fields and foraging bees which live in the figments of my imagination, my earnest celebration of honeybees' value to mankind, my heartfelt gratitude towards their laborious work, and my rallying cry to protect and save them from the devastating colony collapse disorder.

I so love these thoughts of honey and bees, and hope you will too. Each time I read again, they put on a smile on my face and nudge a few nods on my head, and I wish that for you too.

"Honey & I" is dedicated to:

1. All who love to join me in the celebration of honey bees and their golden treasures, as there will be so much joy and pleasure in immediately recognising so many delightful truths.

2. Everyone who is curious about honey and bees, as there will be such a great sense of gratification and enlightenment from discovering many precious truths never known before.

DAY 1

This marvels me to depths - that only God himself can intend how good honey it is to be and fashion the flowers and bees to perfect it; neither the most ingenious mind nor the most cutting-edge science can fathom it or produce it.

DAY 2

A blob of honey a day banishes the bug away.

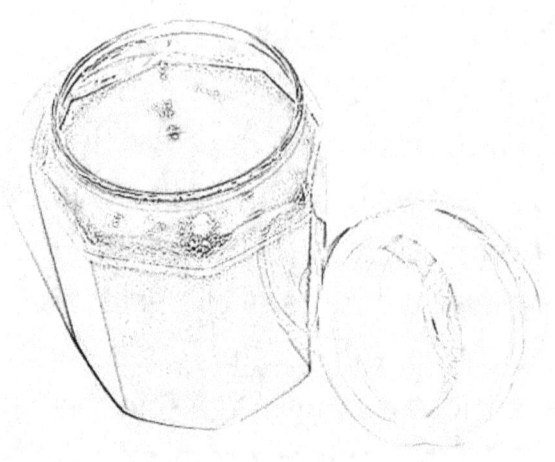

DAY 3

—◦∽∾◦—

See your health index rise as you
upgrade from processed table sugar
to this all natural multivitamin,
honey.

DAY 4

Honey is glistening liquid gold, filled with health nuggets only the buzzing insect can deposit.

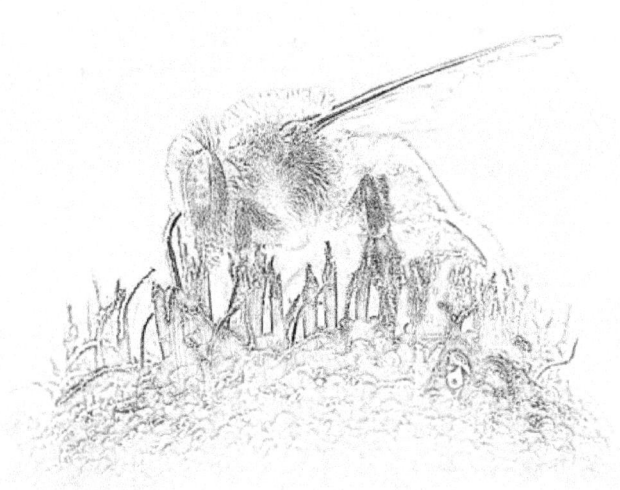

DAY 5

The reverberation of honey benefits will change the way people talk about honey and experience honey, turning consumption into a special ceremony, and with its own special tastes, honey will find a new star status as a chic and awe-inspiring golden liquid.

DAY 6

Eating for health has never been sweeter.

DAY 7

Discover how incredibly intelligent natural honey is, why this super-food must be differentiated from other sweeteners, and how it can bring a slew of amazing health benefits and spin-offs to your life and the lives of your loved ones.

DAY 8

Excellent in any weight reduction plan, honey produces more energy than its weight and in the process uses part of our accumulated fat and cholesterol.

DAY 9

Tell your little ones that honey doesn't come from the bears or the factories, but from the stomach of nectar-collecting bees.

DAY 10

Today medical research is turning in more and more evidence of honey's importance as a healing food, placing the natural sweetener way above its already fascinating status as a kitchen ingredient and folklore medicine.

DAY 11

Considering its healing power, energy-giving buzz and ambrosial sweetness, this sticky liquid made from flowers by bees deserves a much more elevated status that reflects its worth.

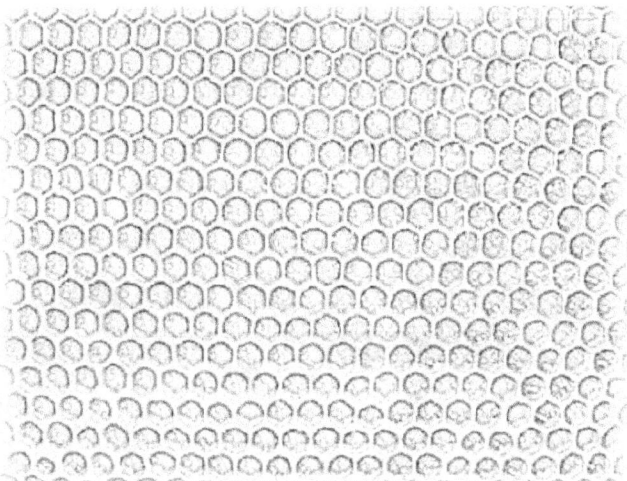

DAY 12

I believe the best labs can create synthetic liquids that look and taste like real honey and even have the same glucose-fructose molecular structure, but NEVER can they fake something that works the same as real honey for our health and well-being. Because the bees have added a MYSTERIOUS GOODNESS of their own that can never be comprehended by the most ingenious mind or counterfeited by the most advanced technology.

DAY 13

—∙⚬⚭⚬∙—

Parents, be informed on the effects of different sugars and take action. No one is going to care and plan more for your family's health than you, not the schools, not the food authorities, and not the doctors. I believe honey can help us and the future generations turn away from refined HFCS and the host of harmful artificial sweeteners that are wreaking much havoc on the human body. Pass the word around about what the bees have given us, convert as many of your friends and loved ones as possible before they get whirled into the confusing and deceptive world of sugars.

DAY 14

―――∞C∞∞――――

Let's celebrate the goodness of honey and the work of the giver, the honeybees.

DAY 15

―――∞C∞∞――――

I strongly believe that honey is more than just the sum of its sugars; the honeybees have added something special inside that cannot be mimicked by any artificial sugars.

DAY 16

Why don't I ask doctors if honey is good for diabetics? The problem is, too many doctors take an emotive stance on sugar and an ill-informed view about alternative medicine. And anyway, since when did they take a good interest in how natural food can heal our natural body?

DAY 17

Why won't I agree with dieticians who say reducing the intake of refined sugar is as good as not adding honey to the diet? Because honey is more than a sweetener! Its healthful benefits go well beyond its sweet qualities!

DAY 18

Please don't misunderstand me again. I'm certainly not trying to get you binge wilfully on this sweet. I am talking about choosing honey over other sugars and eating it for health. "Not all fats are equal" seems to be common knowledge for people who are dieting and weight conscious, but "all sugars are not created equal" sometimes seems to come across as bizarre and counter intuitive. People need to know that there are good sugar, bad sugar and even dangerous sugar! There are so many guises of sweeteners, and some come in names that you can even pronounce!

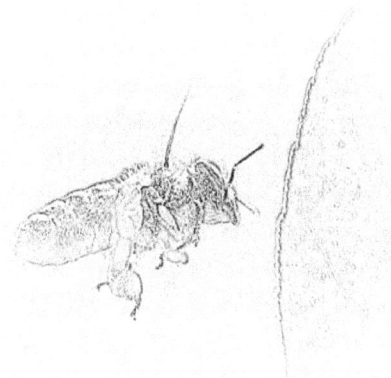

DAY 19

Did you see the reflection on the glassy golden liquid? The lushest mountain meadow bursting with the most aromatic wildflowers and the opulence of therapeutic scents, and with the foraging honeybees sucking the spirit of the healing plants under the happiest sunshine.

DAY 20

Honey, calories imbued with rich natural goodness that only the buzzing six-legged insect can give.

DAY 21

If you can't tolerate the taste of honey, don't give up on this super-food, because no one type of honey tastes alike and chances are you haven't tried enough of the different floral varietals to find one that your taste buds will really adore. Keep exploring, I'm too certain that you will find at least one favorite varietal that you will love for life.

DAY 22

—◦∾◦—

Our body needs a daily influx of vitamins and minerals to ward off invaders. What better way than to partake in delicious honey?

DAY 23

—◦∾◦—

Conversations about honey are changing. With more and more evidence of honey medical benefits turning up in all directions, the golden liquid has dropped its image of an old-fashioned and mundane commodity and is on its way to gaining a chic and awe-inspiring star status.

DAY 24

———◇○◇◇◇○◇———

Eat only 100% pure, unadulterated honey. Beware of any added ingredients like HFCF, karo syrup, maltodextrin, isoglucose, dextrin, multidextrose, novelose, and many other unpronounceable chemicals. Remember: Pure honey has NO other ingredients.

DAY 25

———◇○◇◇◇○◇———

For me eating honey is not just a positive emotional response that my taste buds elicit but a smart decision my mind makes to gain from this intelligent food.

DAY 26

Honey is far from being a mundane, humdrum commodity. Its flavor, viscosity, color are a fascinating snapshot of its source; a complex combination of factors including floral crops and flower sources, bee species, landscape, climate, weather conditions, season, amount of rainfall and sunshine, and soil chemistry. Cast aside all superficialities and let the mind conceive the depths of its riches.

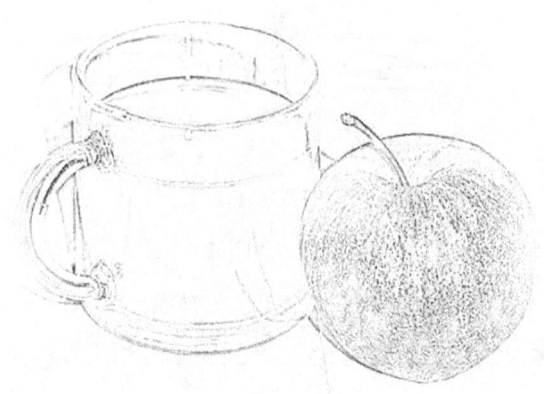

DAY 27

D.C. Jarvis in his book "Folk Medicine" (1958) recommended apple cider vinegar as a powerful alternative medicine that could destroy harmful bacteria in the digestive tract, and advised that adding honey to apple cider vinegar would enhance the healing power of the vinegar. He called the tonic *Honegar*.

DAY 28

—◇○◇◇○◇—

Have a strep throat? Pop a small
piece of honeycomb into the mouth,
chew it like a gum. Soothes and
remedies faster than any lozenges.

DAY 29

—◇○◇◇○◇—

I can't disagree more that honey has
a few positive health effects that
have been studied a little bit.

DAY 30

——◦◦❦◦◦——

God *loves* all his creations, but I tend to believe there are particular creatures that he *likes*, and the bee is one of them. He has given the TINY insect such a BIG role that's so wonderfully and intimately enmeshed in the needs of us mankind.

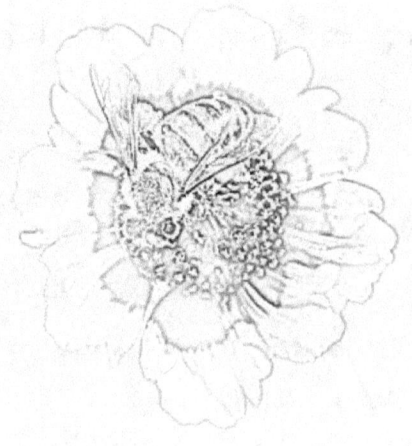

DAY 31

Many people had doubts if Albert Einstein had really made this bold speculation, "if the bee disappeared off the surface of the globe, man would have only four years to live". But the fact is the honey bees are responsible for pollinating a third of global farm and these foods provide a significant intake of our daily calories, minerals, vitamins, and anti-oxidants, can we say with certainty that our world would not face an ecology apocalypse without the bees?

DAY 32

I'm grateful how science has pointed to the goodness in honey, but I'm more amazed by the way Mother Nature has intended the sweet composition to benefit our human bodies.

DAY 33

I see the honey hibernation diet as neither a mystical cure nor hype. It is not intended as a magic diet or one-time programme, but a way of life based on good science, followed in conjunction with a healthy lifestyle to derive far reaching health benefits.

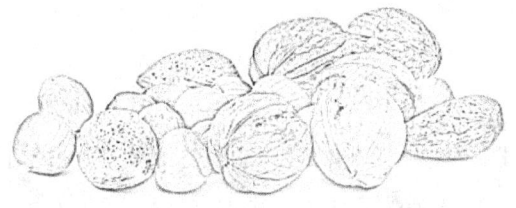

DAY 34

Listen to the honeybee buzz in the blossom-laden fields; they are announcing the beginning of a busy day. Behold the pollen-dusted honeybees latched on the nectaries; they are sucking the sweetest liquid to fill their honey tummies. Consider how the bees zip from flower to flower to pollinate the plants, causing their ovaries to swell into succulent fruits, and then into crunchy nuts. Tell the world to save the dying bees, because without them, it would be a life too unimaginable.

DAY 35

After two years of eating honey daily before bedtime, I got out of a chronic adrenal fatigue condition and asthmatic cough that dogged me since I was a child. That's why I can't speak highly enough of this bee food.

DAY 36

Why do I avoid honey in my conversation with doctors? Because far too many of them are too quick to tell me that honey is just sugar, sugar is sugar, and sugar is bad for me. They can't be more wrong than this, can they?

DAY 37

Yes, honey is a sugar but one that is supremely healthier than the refined and artificial.

DAY 38

Research studies and evidence on honey benefits are pouring in from all over the world. If they are but a bunch of hoopla to you, then listen to what real people who have no strings attached to you, have to say about their experience and the wonders of honey.

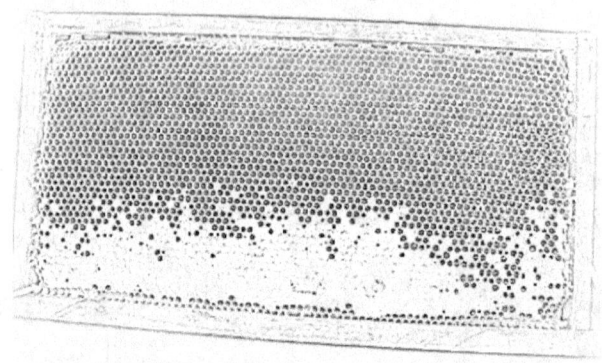

DAY 39

—◦∽◦—

Why do I like an old-timey, grandmother food like natural honey? Because I haven't got the slightest conviction that the new, modern, chemical-laden synthetic foods could be of any good.

DAY 40

Since the beginning of time, honey has been prized for its medicinal qualities and ability to heal coughs and wounds. Honey was food fit for the gods by the Greeks and Romans, an essential in burial vaults for the Egyptian pharaohs, and a rejuvenating power in the skin care regime of the legendary beauty, Cleopatra. There is something enduring about honey, impervious to the pull of trend-chasing and commercialism. Forever, our love affair with this timeless food will endure.

DAY 41

If it's so easy for people to agree that not all fats are equal; there are good fats and bad fats, I just can't see why it is so difficult for people to accept that not all sugars are equal and that there are good sugars and bad sugars too.

DAY 42

I hear the advice "Say no to sugar" often enough. But why? I would say "Say no to bad sugars"!

DAY 43

The doctors never fail to tell us that our body is unable to utilize refined sugars which are void of all nutrients and our body tissues in fact must relinquish precious vitamins and minerals to detoxify and eliminate them from our system, which often leads to nutrient deficiencies and the gradual deterioration of our cells and organs. But did they ever tell you once that our body needs some sugar, and good sugar, honey ideally, can provide a positive supply of liver glycogen for healthy effects of brain metabolism?

DAY 44

I can't help feeling excited by the prospect of how many more people would give up refined and artificial sweeteners and turn to natural honey when they realise its restorative power during sleep can actually reduce incidences of hypertension, diabetes, cardiovascular disease, stroke, cancer, arthritis and many other related diseases.

DAY 45

⸻∘◦❍◦∘⸻

I saw and felt with my own senses how a dab of honey took away the throbbing pain from my soup-scalded hand in just a few minutes and eventually left no redness, blister, or any sign of burn on the skin after half an hour.

DAY 46

⸻∘◦❍◦∘⸻

I'm not fanatical, but just true and honest about honey can do that most doctors and dieticians don't tell you.

DAY 47

I was troubled by a painful nose staph for several weeks until I smeared a drop of honey on the infection. It was all cleared in two days, with just three applications. Time and again, honey has wowed me.

DAY 48

Is there even a need to persevere in sticking to taking a spoonful of honey before bedtime? It's probably the easiest daily health regime around.

DAY 49

The link between quality sleep and body immunity isn't that obvious to me until I start eating honey at bedtime and I learn that honey facilitates the release of the wellness hormone, melatonin in my body, stocks my liver with glycogen, and fuels my brain adequately to prevent metabolic stress.

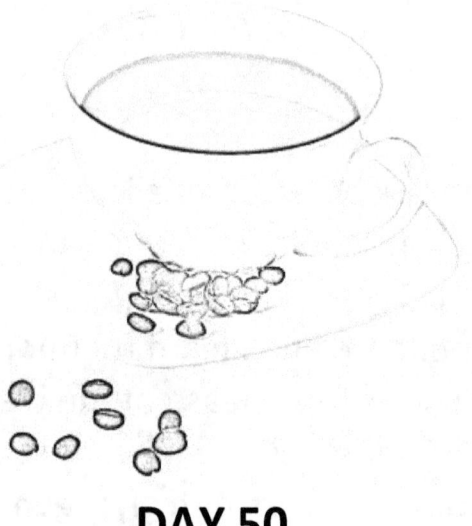

DAY 50

I believe the successful marketing of honey as an additive in chocolates, cereals, tea, energy drinks, fruits and nuts is not just a result of advertising ingenuity, but a growing body of scientific confirmation of what our grandmothers and great-grandmothers had believed all their lives.

DAY 51

It has been shown over and over again that honey suppresses children's cough reflex at night more effectively than pharmacy-dispensed Dextromethorphan. I believe this has much to do with its unique ability to naturally induce deep sleep.

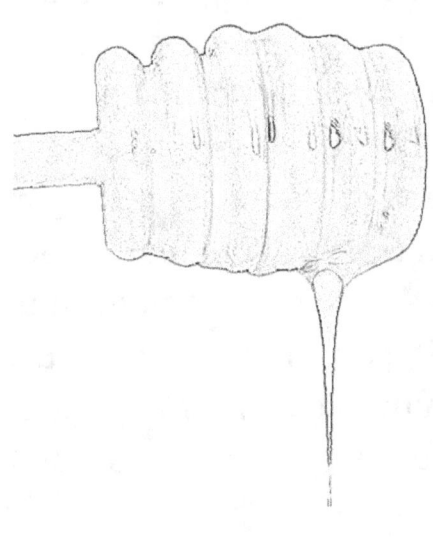

DAY 52

How often do we hear these erroneous statements being made, and even many times from the medical profession? "Honey is water super-saturated with sugar. You got to be kidding yourself if you tell me that it is healthier than any other concentrated sugar product. Sugar is sugar; people eat it because it is a carbohydrate rich in energy. It doesn't matter where it comes from, the cane or the bees, costing more doesn't make it any better. So, do not be so naive and delude yourself, the liquid from the bees is just as fattening like any other sugars and can cause problems like obesity and diabetes. It contains traces of amino acids, vitamins, and minerals but the

amount is so insignificant that you
need to eat tons of it to benefit from
it."

DAY 53

Don't underestimate the healthful
enzymes in bee food. They may be
minute in quantity, but overtime,
when consumed daily and
consistently, they can spin off
powerful accumulative effects in our
health immune function and a great
sense of wellness that is huge
enough to be felt and seen.

DAY 54

The medicinal properties and anti-viral qualities that enable the plants to survive and resist the attacks of microbes and insects, already pre-exist in the nectar that the bees collect. The bees just enhance them.

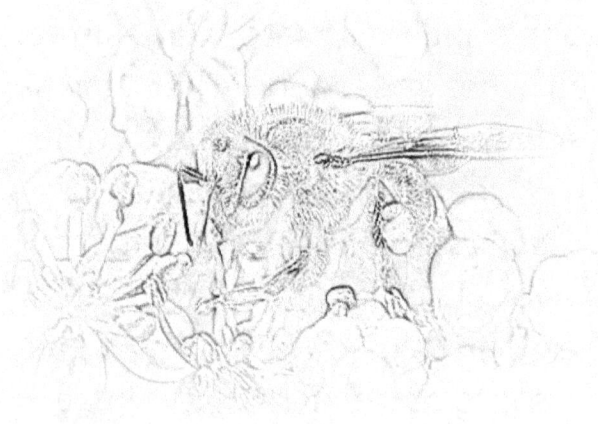

DAY 55

What's the point of lamenting over the prevalence of toxic-forming sugars in our foods and fake honey in the market? We are often sad about facing the uncertainties of eating harmful sugars and buying adulterated honey, but not enough to make enquiries on their source and origin or do anything to avoid them.

DAY 56

Two reasons why I've never referred to honey as *bee vomit* even through it's helpful in explaining the honey-making process especially to the kids. One, it turns people off. Second, it's not true. Honey is a result of the bee's purposeful regurgitation, which is the bringing up of desirable nutrients voluntarily, whereas vomiting is the involuntary spew of repulsive matter.

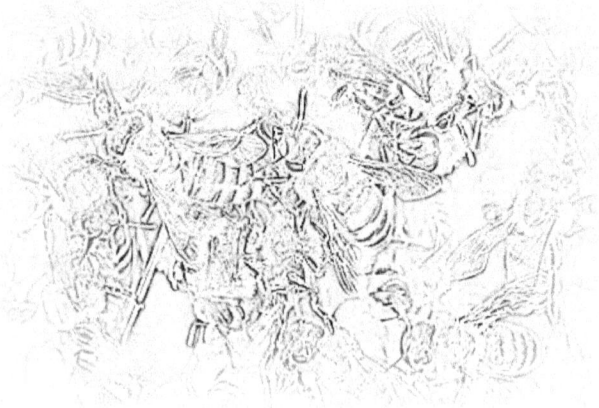

DAY 57

It is a *fact* that the rapid wipe-out of bee colonies is alarming and presenting an overwhelming threat to the food chain, but why is it not getting the same attention from governments and activists as for the global warming *theory*? The reason is clear, but unfathomable.

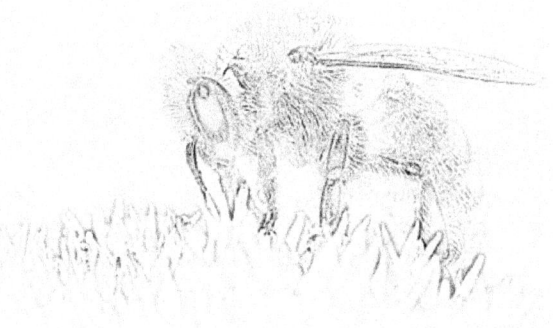

DAY 58

Our pollinating friends are under stress; please help them to move on.

DAY 59

I love to think that consuming a teaspoonful of honey and bee pollen was a daily regimen of Fred Harold Hale, world's oldest man (1890-2004, Guinness World Records).

DAY 60

—◦◦◦—

I bet Hippocrates, father of medicine (431 B.C) had a pot of honey in his mind when he proclaimed "Let food be thy medicine and medicine be thy food."

DAY 61

—◦◦◦—

See how much more you would love honey when you see the glob of the golden treasure you place on your palate as the beautiful life work of thousands of honeybees earnestly performing their foraging rituals in the blossoming fields.

DAY 62

You have to know this, like any foods, not all honey is created equal. It is not difficult to find expensive fake, adulterated honey out there, but it's just impossible to get pure, quality honey at the same low price as corn syrup!

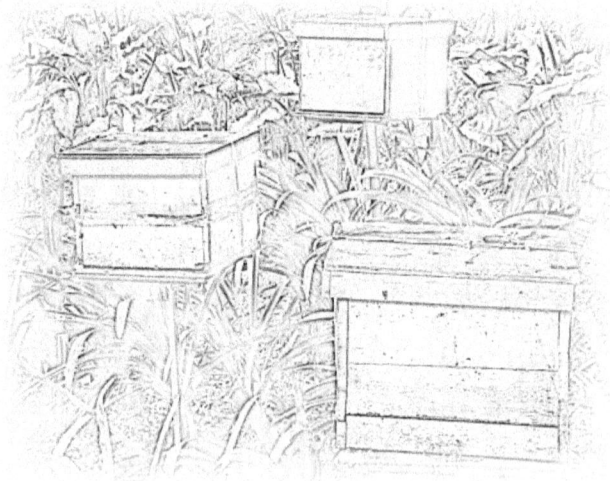

DAY 63

—◇○◇◇○◇—

We all know that it's an impossible task to test from home if the honey you buy is pure. But ah-ha! You can test the beekeeper on how he/she has obtained that jar of honey for you!

DAY 64

—◇○◇◇○◇—

The association between honey and medicine is too far-fetched? Not at all when it is personally experienced.

DAY 65

Be wise, "pure honey" label doesn't necessarily mean 100% pure honey as it only suggests the presence of pure honey in unknown quantity, and "local honey" doesn't always guarantee honey produced locally as it may only mean imported honey packed locally.

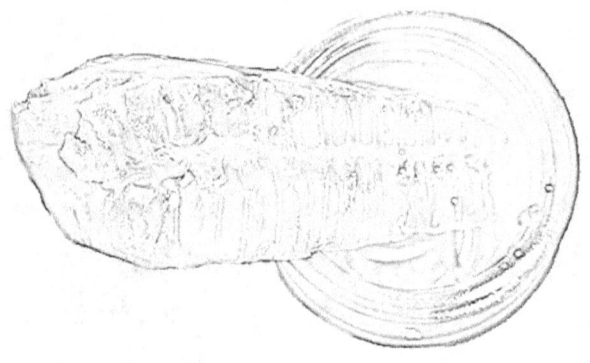

DAY 66

—————⊸∘᯽⊙∘⊶—————

Seriously, I think you don't have to
be a honey aficionado to tell if the
honey is smooth, woody, bold or
earthy. This may sound offensive to
the honey connoisseurs, but eating
honey is really so much more
straightforward than tasting wine.

DAY 67

—————⊸∘᯽⊙∘⊶—————

It would be too cool to own a chain
of honey bars all over my country,
where people can come and sample
the different kinds of honey from
around the world.

DAY 68

There is an incredible, addictive sense of satisfaction, the more I write, the deeper my conviction became and the more I felt I could help others discover honey.

DAY 69

Honey is far more than a tasty treat. Loaded with healing and therapeutic properties, it is nature's tonic for a healthier, stronger human body.

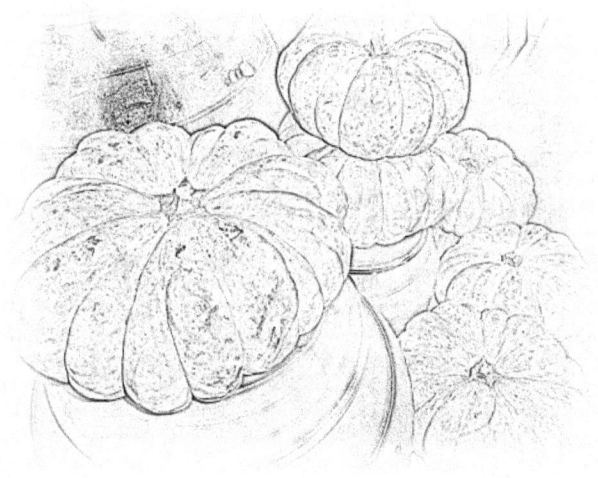

DAY 70

I have after all I enjoyed so much of this natural sweetener, how can I not be grateful to its giver - the honeybees, the silent hero, master pollinator of our flowering plants and crops!

DAY 71

Have nothing to do with greedy beekeepers. The love of money and the commitment to upholding quality and safety standards of honey seldom go hand-in-hand.

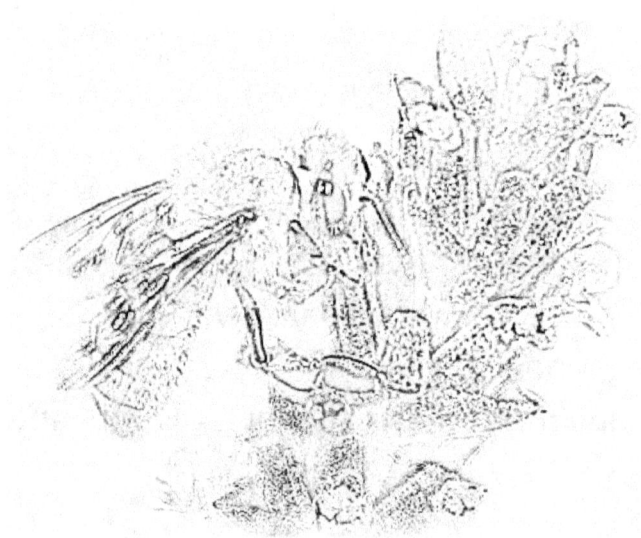

DAY 72

Nothing else tastes quite like pure honey. There are countless delicious artificial sweeteners made by Big Pharma, but nothing has come close to honey.

DAY 73

If you haven't tasted honey direct from the hive, you haven't quite tasted honey.

DAY 74

Did I hear that honey is a mundane and boring food? How would you like it to be? Mellow and smooth, bold and woody, dark and cloying, light but refreshing, earthy and overpowering, exotic with calming notes, vibrant and aromatic, warm and spicy, mildly floral, sensual with a hint of nutty aftertaste, a touch of citrus, pleasing and authentic? Sorry I can't stop, but I have to tell you that the bees can produce them all!

DAY 75

Do you see the mercenary corruptibility of the human species? Honey is too weak in attracting the same kind of research funding as conventional medicines because the powerful medicinal qualities it possesses cannot be patented. So, its beneficial applications in diseases and ailments remain largely unexplored by the masses.

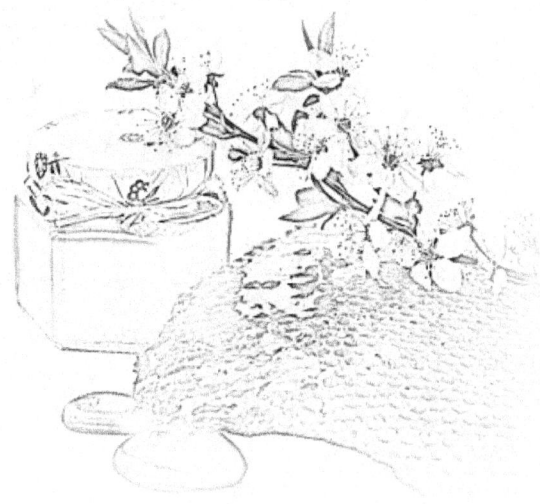

DAY 76

If you tell doctors that you use anti-bacterial honey to treat burns and cuts, they would be quick to rebut that bacteria can't grow in any sugar concentrated environment and honey isn't a special exception. But they have forgotten (or have no inkling at all) that the bees have included something "extra" from their own to incredibly avoid or reduce scarring and inflammation and bring about healing of wounds much more speedily.

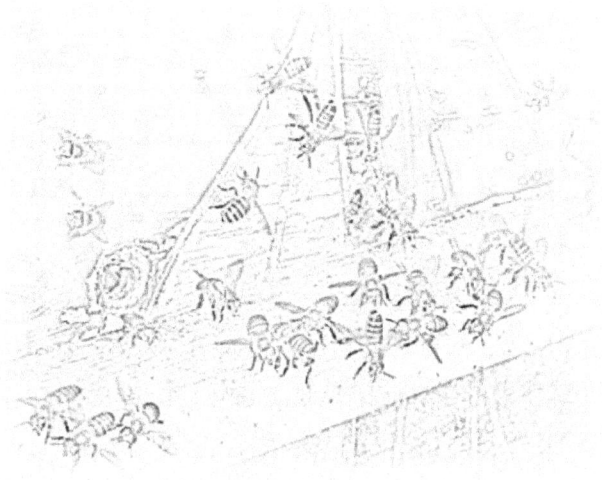

DAY 77

—◇○◇○◇—

We can't deny the bees are getting more attention than other creepy crawlies or any of the insects that sting, like wasps and hornets. The bees seem to have an indescribable allure in them, an almost divine and mysterious charm that endears people to think and talk much about them.

● ● ●

DAY 78

Some ingredients in Traditional Chinese Medicine remedies are said to have the unique ability of multiplying the concoctions' healing effects many times over. I am not surprised to find honey to be one of them.

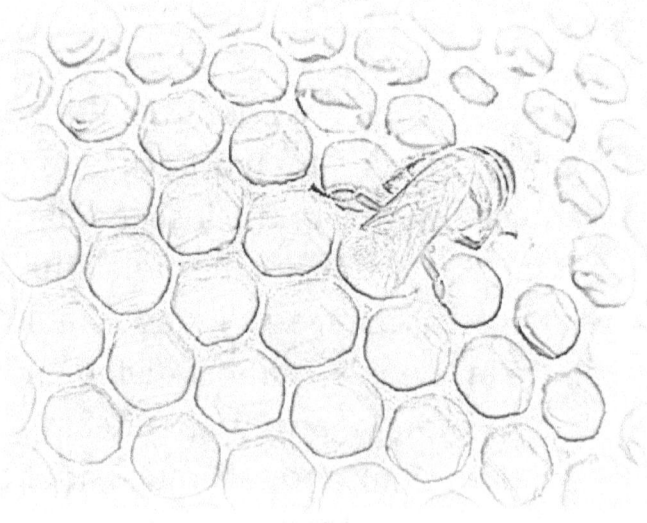

DAY 79

⌥

Shall we the big-brained humans ever comprehend how the bee has all these figured out with its grass seed-sized brain – process memory of hundreds of flower sources and distinguish their scents, calculate complex foraging flights and navigate the shortest route between flowers, measure time by the sun, ensure adequate fuel for their journey, and communicate to other bees the direction and quality of a food source?

DAY 80

Why do so many still continue to use refined and artificial sugars instead of honey when they know very well how toxic they can be? Well, because knowledge is not the same as wisdom.

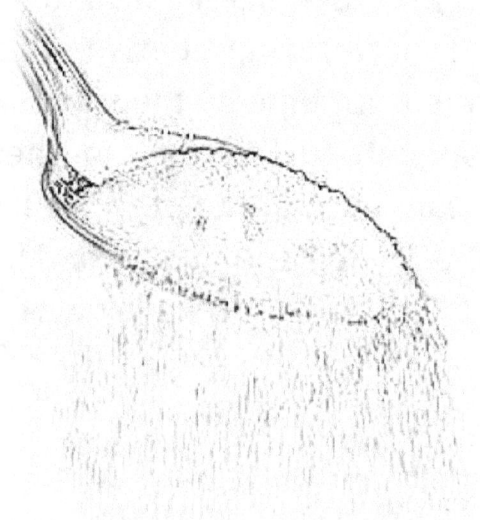

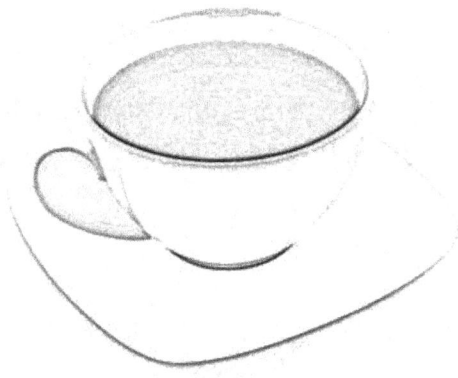

DAY 81

If you are going to add sugar to your tea or coffee anyway, you might as well add one that is capable of doing some good to your body, like honey.

DAY 82

Honey, you're my sweetest, most trusted and natural choice for life!

DAY 83

After two years of having honey on my kitchen table, I was happy to clean out my medicine cabinet piled up with expired over-the-counter medical supplies including throat lozenges, cough formula Dextromethorphan, antihistamines, Paracetamol tablets, Burnaid gel, and antiseptic cream. And now I'm more than contented with having no need to replenish the cabinet with new ones.

DAY 84

Great, science is now playing catch-up on the implications honey has on liver health and sleep quality, the healing benefits of honey that our predecessors had experienced centuries ago. Let's hope that conventional medicine will eventually take the blinders off to recognize that honey has been too grossly underutilized.

DAY 85

A safer and more natural remedy than any sleeping pill, honey facilitates the release of melatonin, the "wellness hormone" in our brain to give us restorative sleep.

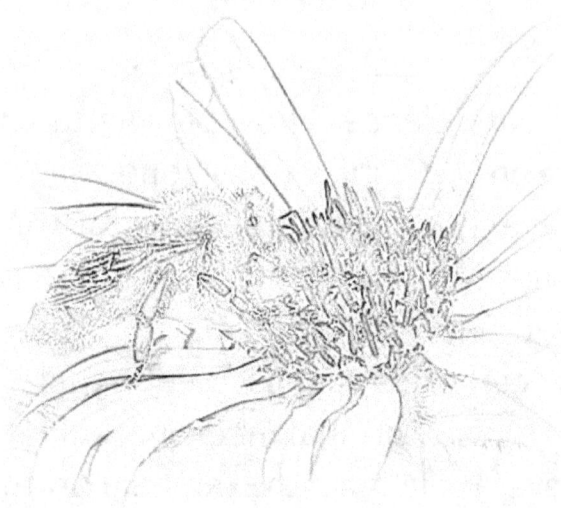

DAY 86

—◦∽∾◦—

I eat sugar made from the delicately
scented, pretty frilly flowers resting
in faraway meadows that only the
tiny yellow and black striped fairies
can find.

DAY 87

The ancient Egyptian remedy for cataracts is one of the most mind-blowing healing benefits of honey that even modern people of today can vouch for: apply a few drops of raw honey directly to the eyes. Honestly, when I first read about it, it sounded too jeopardous. But when more people start to write to me and share about their own experience of using honey to "dissolve" cataracts, cure dry eyes, freshen eyes, and prevent eye strains, I figure that if we can readily accept chemical-loaded prescription solutions, perhaps a natural eye drop shouldn't be that mind-shattering after all.

DAY 88

Raw honey, a one-ingredient natural face wash made from flowers by bees – gentle, moisturizing, and antiseptic. Daily, smear honey on your face, leave it for 5 minutes and rinse off. Try it if you haven't. It's surprisingly effective.

DAY 89

I never knew how my favorite tonic, honey woke up my sluggish liver and turned my health around until I read about its 1:1 balance of glucose and fructose that makes it the most ideal food to form a liver glycogen supply, the primary fuel reserve for the brain in human metabolism.

DAY 90

I am happy not to explore the myriad of empty-calorie and caffeine-loaded energy drinks in the super marts. I am already getting my superb, natural blast of energy from my ten-second home concoction - honey and water.

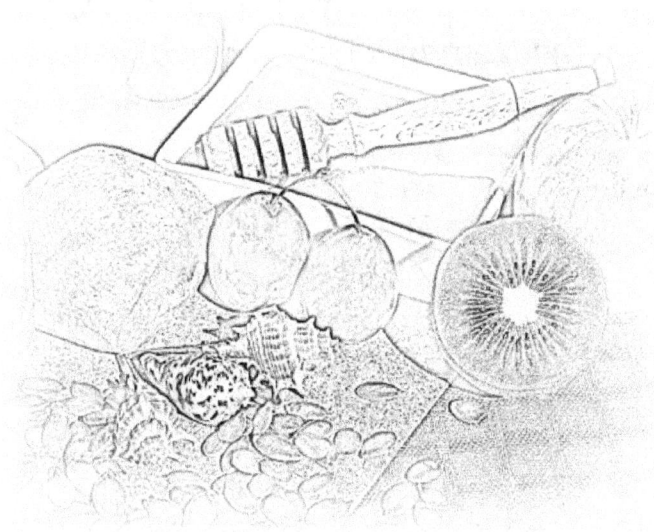

DAY 91

Yes, I do fully understand that no one food can be excessively eaten without compromising your health and also do completely recognise that no single food can determine the state of your health than your overall diet. But still, I do not see why I should be in any way downplaying the tremendously positive health benefits honey can have in our living.

DAY 92

—◦◦◦—

This morning's local papers report that "adverse reactions to a conventional medicine do not necessarily mean that the medicine is harmful, all medicines can cause adverse reactions, but many are considered safe as the benefits outweighs the risks". This is plain sloppy research at best or outright disingenuous at worse? How many of such risks are immediately visible? And since when has *safe* been defined as having more benefits than risks? So what does that make of alternative medicine like bee pollen, propolis, and honey? Why are they granted so little recognition in the medical field? Too safe?

DAY 93

Struggling with a sluggish liver? Mike and Stuart McInnes in The Hibernation diet advise eating honey. Its 1:1 ratio of glucose and fructose makes it the most ideal food to form a liver glycogen, the primary fuel reserve for the brain in human metabolism.

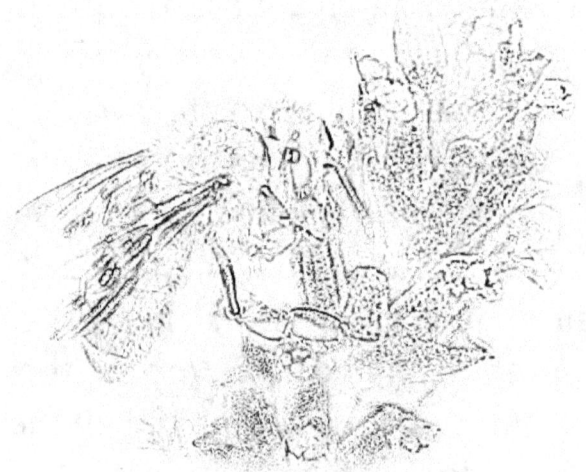

DAY 94

―――――∞◦ᏫᏯᏫ◦∞―――――

I remember honeybees were an everyday sight in my school when I was about seven. They were everywhere in the compound, the field, and even the canteen. But as the years went by, with the country's burgeoning population and rapid urbanisation, it became harder and harder to encounter the bees. Today, they seem to have flat-out disappeared.

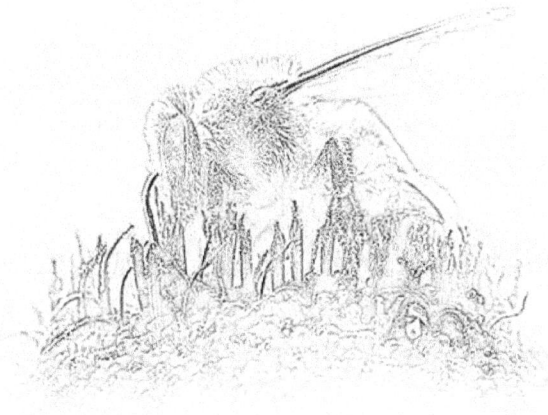

DAY 95

I'm fortunate to be spared from the troubles of seasonal allergies of flower pollens here. But the frequency of receiving testimonies from those living abroad constrains me to put this impressive benefit of eating honey on record – "Raw local honey effectively relieves seasonal allergies: 1-3 teaspoons per day, either straight or mixed into beverage or other foods".

DAY 96

I eat honey to think better, exercise better, and sleep better.

DAY 97

Shame on those greedy farmers who are destroying bee colonies for the fear they would abscond with the honey, clipping off the wings of queen bees to prevent them from swarming, taking away all the bees' honey and feeding them only sugar syrup, causing honey contamination with their use of synthetic pesticides and antibiotics to combat pests. Honest beekeepers really don't deserve the same rotten image anti-honey groups have of the beekeeping trade.

DAY 98

—◦∾⧜∾◦—

Raw honey is a great natural source of prebiotics that help beneficial bacteria or probiotics grow and flourish in our digestive system. No wonder so many have attested that it works like a charm for heartburns, flatulence, and abdominal cramps.

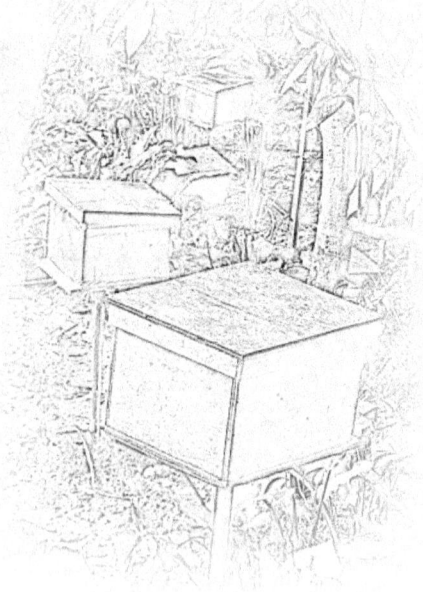

DAY 99

I prescribe to the world's sweetest antibiotic that is least costly, all natural and free of harmful side-effects - honey.

DAY 100

I like to have cream or thick honey twirled around the end of a chop-stick like a candy. It wanes all the urges for chocolate bars, ice-cream, and wafers. My favourite way of combating sugar cravings and binges!

DAY 101

Foreigners cannot imagine the place I live and some have not heard of it. Buy local honey, they advise. But I live in an urban food dessert where bee farms are extinct. Visit the countryside, they coax. I would love to but there isn't one. Love the bees, they urged. Sure, but I hardly see any bees here, in fact they are treated as pests. Become an urban backyard beekeeper, they quip. That would be a dream come true, but beekeeping is not lawful here. You're probably the most unlikely person on earth to celebrate the bees and their honey. Yes, I think so, but I guess people yearn for what they lack most.

Epilogue

The benefits of honey are amazing - as an excellent source of energy, antioxidants, and vitamins, for beautiful hair and skin, weight loss, healing of burns, cuts and wounds, liver health, digestion, building immunity, treatment of sore throats, flu, insomnia, etc. The more frequently people talk about them, the more I believe that the status of honey has to be elevated to more than just a sweetener or a kitchen condiment.

It's said that the average honey bee will actually make only one twelfth of a teaspoon of honey in its lifetime and it takes about 550 honey bees to make 1 pound of honey (that is, less than half a kilogram) from some 2 million flowers. So, appreciate and enjoy every bit of the bees' hard work for you.

Wishing you many sweet discoveries in life!

About The Author

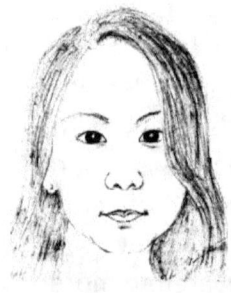 Ruth Tan is the founder of http://www.benefits-of-honey.com, the number one ranked website on Google, Yahoo! and Bing for benefits of honey and an immensely rich, quality resource on honey and its benefits, and a plethora of health-related issues. Growing everyday with more and more people from all over the world sharing with her health benefits of honey through the website is her conviction that honey is able to make a remarkable difference in the health of this generation and the generations to come.

She is also the author of the books "Darling, Honey is Good for You!" and "How to Effectively Use Honey as Medicine: What Doctors Don't Tell You."

Random Thoughts III, Attack of the Inquisitive Mind

by Leland Hoburg

10423092

Conservative, Moderate, or Liberal, all are
politicians

I am not running for office but if I was
here are more thoughts on the process...

It is that time of year again, when the
political debates start up, the primaries get
rolling, the candidates are out kissing babies and
shaking hands, and labels are being bandied
about like weapons. Are you a Conservative,
Moderate, or Liberal? Does it really matter? All
are politicians looking to fill a niche to get votes
and be elected, but in the end, they are all
politicians. What would be truly refreshing
would be someone to label themselves as a
patriot, an independent, free of political party
affiliations. Would they be elected? Who knows,
as long as their platform seems reasonable and
presented in a logical manner, again who knows.

1

I would like to someone run on a platform of term limits, campaign finance reform, and further limits on special interests and lobbyist. If someone actually proposed these ideas, the other candidates would label them as socialist or communist because they sound anti-American but they are what America truly needs. The President said it himself, there is a disconnect between those politicians in Washington D.C. and the rest of the country. Labels are powerful in the political arena, labels define who you are, who your adversaries are, and who your allies are, and in large part where you stand on the issues of the day. Another thing I would like to see is the end of attack ads against other candidates, if you do not have something nice to say do not say anything at all. Last refreshing thought, a candidate who takes no money from special interest groups and limits all contributions to no more than fifty dollars. Part of the reform process would have to come from the media and news outlets by offering free advertising space to all candidates regardless of affiliation, but hey, there is big money is political season advertising.

If I were to run for Office

First of all, why does anyone want to run for office? Several simple reasons:

- Job security, it is nearly impossible to vote out incumbents unless they do something drastically wrong or there is a massive shift in public open.

- Great benefits, at least on the state and federal level, the best that tax payers can buy.

- The best perks that lobbyist can buy.

- Lastly, at least at the federal level, an easy workweek, think of this, last year both houses of congress were actually only in session eighty days, which is only sixteen weeks of work out of fifty-two. By comparison, the average U.S. worker worked fifty-one weeks in 2011, mostly due to the higher amount of "part time" employees who work without benefits.

So what would my platform be? The platform is education reform, job creation through small business and local economies of scale, campaign finance reform and congressional term limits. I would focus on these issues, leaving alone abortion (until the Supreme Court says otherwise is legal and no man has any right to tell a woman otherwise), gay marriage or civil unions are doing well on their own and gaining momentum, taxes are an old and tired song, redistribution of wealth will get you laughed off the stage, reducing redundancy in government is the equivalent killing the golden goose, improvement of social services and reducing waste in the system is another golden egg that is off limits, and immigration reform which is another tired old song.

- Education reform, how is this going to work and why do we need it? Let me start with a few anecdotes on our education system. A few years ago I read a Bill Wundrum column on an eighth grade graduation test that several of us read and determined (all of us had advanced degrees) that we would be hard pressed to pass certain portions of the test. Add in to this a test booklet we found cleaning out my great aunts house; she was a schoolteacher in one of the last one-room schoolhouses in Illinois, of similar design and complexity. My father, who was still teaching at the time, said the test was harder than the G.E.D. test at the time. A sad note on the dumbing down of America, and the decline of our prominence in the world as the bastion of higher learning and innovation, consider this, Japan graduates more engineers from its universities than any other nation whereas the U.S. graduates more lawyers then the rest of the G20 combined. At one time an eighth grade diploma meant you could find a job and provide for your family, a high school diploma was an automatic entry into a factory job, a bachelors degree meant you could teach your area of expertise to primary and secondary students, a masters enabled you to teach at a community college, and a doctoral degree meant you could do research and teach at a university. As we have progressed we have done away with the eighth grade graduation, a high school diploma or equivalent qualifies you for manual labor and non management service industry jobs, a bachelors means you are trainable, a masters means you can teach, and a doctoral means you can do research. So how would I reform education? There are three basic steps to the reformation of our education system. One, do away with standardized testing with the exception of the ACT and SAT, which are used for college admission, more time is spent in the classroom teaching to perform on whatever state test is being used. Students should be able to pass knowledge test at three points in a student's primary and secondary education career, at eighth grade including knowledge of the state constitution, in high school passing a U.S. constitution test, and after the sophomore year to see if the student is ready to graduate and progress on to a community college or university. At this point students will have two options, to continue to prepare for a university or to begin learning a trade skill. If this sounds similar to a European educational system then you are right, too many students graduate high school without any marketable skills and are fit only for minimum wage slave jobs in fast food and big box retail.

- Job creation through small business and local economies of scale, small business is the backbone of our economy, part of this is reforming the tax code to make it more lucrative to be an owner operator by raising the income level where taxes are to be collected thus leaving more money in the pockets of the working class. No taxes collected until income passes sixty-thousand dollars per person or one-hundred-thousand dollars for a family or small business. By putting money back into the pockets of the working class you have the opportunity to increase the amount of disposable income moving through the economy and by focusing on the local businesses you put money back into U.S. business and not into large multinational companies that may or may not keep that money here in the U.S.A. I am not xenophobic but charity starts at home before it goes abroad.

- Campaign finance reform and congressional term limits, are actually easy, simply put a limit on the amount of money that can be raised and spent, eliminate political action groups, limit campaign donations to one-hundred dollars per individual or group, and eliminate political parties all candidates stand on their own platform not some amorphous political parties platform catering to the fringes to appease the middle. Term limits are also easy, limit the time a person can serve in congress to twenty years of total time between both houses. It should be a sign that term limits are necessary when the average age of a senator is over sixty-five, an age when most people are retiring from work and not looking to extend their career another six years. We have term limits on the President, some states have term limits for their governor, and some cities have term limits for their mayor, why then are we afraid to set term limits for congress. Our founding fathers never envisioned a member of congress dying in office due to extreme old age and serving over forty years in office. What our founding fathers envisioned were civic-minded gentleman landowners as senators and representatives, giving a short period of public service for the betterment of the country, not professional politicians giving an entire adult lifetime of service for the betterment of their pockets. Is it sad that of the top ten wealthiest members of

congress, nine of them are democrats
including the number one spot.

What prevents me from running for office?
Money, I am not a fortunate one or a millionaires
son. No one who runs for state level or federal
level office does so without deep pockets or deep-
pocketed friends.

First random thoughts of 2012

- It always amazes me at the ignorance people
  display when it comes to technology. I can
  understand people of a certain generation
  having difficulties understanding the
  functionality of technological devices. It is
  the under 50 crowd that always makes me
  shake my head and wonder why some choose
  to remain ignorant and not learn the proper
  applications and uses for current technology.
  The other aspect of this why would you allow
  your child to use the device unsupervised,
  and then blame the company or service when
  your child places charges on your credit card.

As a parent, you have a level of responsibility, a level of required supervision, and a level of educating your child on what is in your beliefs considered acceptable behavior. Blaming a company or service for what your child does is irresponsible on your behalf. Where were you when the child was accessing something you thought they should not? People always assume that what was being accessed is the party to blame. Wrong. Websites cannot "see" who is accessing them, they cannot peer into the mind to see if something is acceptable, and they do not check to see if the person presenting the payment is actually the cardholder. Day in and day out, I hear people whine about how they did not know that "such and such" works a particular way or how a service functions. I have one thing to say: Take time to educate yourself and accept a certain level of responsibility. Ignorance is no excuse, and blaming someone else for your lack of action is the equivalent of "the dog ate my homework." Your lack of responsibility and ignorance does not illicit concern on the part of the customer service personnel, on occasion be an adult and take the blame for your lack of action.

- With the start of the Primaries for the Republican nomination I cannot say this enough, "Who really cares?" both political parties are so out of touch with the average citizen, with the 99%, that watching the political jockeying is almost as entertaining as watching a documentary on the mating habits of the Venezuelan giant slug. Do you want to see real debates, real political discussion, and candidates that the "Joe Average" citizen can associate with then push for reforms in campaign financing by placing limits on fundraising and spending by the candidates, eliminate P.A.C. (Political Action Committees more commonly known as political parties), and eliminate third party political advertising (no more adds by such and such group for political transparency).

- I know I have commented on this before, but outside of LSU and Alabama fans, who cares? The BCS National Title Sham is more fuel for the fire of a playoff system in Division I-A football. After watching great bowl games, particularly the Rose Bowl and the Fiesta Bowl, there were three teams (Wisconsin, Oregon, or Oklahoma State) that should have been playing LSU. All three were conference champions as opposed to Alabama who is not a conference champion. If the game goes again as a low scoring, defensive struggle, and LSU wins again then all that is proven is the first meeting was a clear indicator as to the differences between the two teams, otherwise if Alabama wins it will prove the adage that it is difficult to beat the same team twice in one season. LSU must win for there to be a clear National Champion otherwise both Oregon and OSU have cases for being the BCS champions by virtue of their bowl victories. Enough said, to the NCAA, dump the BCS system, consolidate the 121 D-IA Schools into eight football only conferences, have conference title games, then have an eight-team playoff of conference champions for a true national championship.

It is Just My Opinion...

- Being a curmudgeon is just saying what everyone else is thinking.

- If you are doing things in "God's name" you had better have had direct and verifiable contact along with set of written instructions. Last time this happened, people wandered around the desert for forty years before settling down.

- Why do good people have no luck at all?

- If you tell an OWS protestor to get a job you had better be willing to vacate yours.

- The Bills Of Rights are just that, RIGHTS.

- When did the exercising of your rights become a full contact sport?

- Real life is often stranger than fiction.

- Why is it when you need a little help to get back on your feet people who control that help treat you like second class citizens.

- I may not have much but it is mine and leave it alone.

- Why is it the people who should not reproduce do so like rabbits and those who would be good parents can't?
- When did manners go out of style?
- If you insist on driving under the speed limit in the left lane then you should not be amazed when people tell you that you are number one in sign language.
- I could care less if the NBA never plays again, just another case of the rich arguing over how to get even richer.
- In 1776, acts of civil disobedience sparked a revolution, it can happen again.
- If Politicians were required to work like the average American, our government would run like it should not like it does. Our founding fathers envisioned gentleman congressmen serving for a period of time before retiring to manage their affairs not serving so long as to die while in office.

- I do not want to be President; I want to be a Senator. No term limits, easy hours, and once you are an incumbent great job security.
- Tea party, just another name for pissed off republicans.
- Sanity is only a state of mind.
- Everyone deserves the right to be legally joined in a matrimonial union, so says the Association of Divorce Lawyers, but really, everyone does deserve the chance to be legally joined with that special person.

Quick Notes for New Years Eve, Last Comments of 2011

- NFL and the NBA have labor issues that threaten the season, one phrase: "College Sports," no labor stoppages in the NCAA.
- Bowl season comes and a great variety of games but too many mediocre teams are playing in the bowls.
- Once again the National Title game is a rematch of a regular season game between conference rivals, how boring, and besides

'Bama is not even a conference champion. LSU should be playing OSU, not a conference rival. It is high time for a playoff system.

- It has been a year of big personal changes, new job, new baby, and a new grandbaby on the way.
- As the political year begins in earnest, do we really care who wins in Iowa and New Hampshire. Nothing really matters until the convention is over and we know who the Tea baggers are going to push down our throats. It is time to eliminate political parties; they are the detriment to passing legislation. Our congressional representatives need to vote with the welfare of their constituents in mind and not like lemmings with what their party leaders are saying is the "correct" option.
- Like with computers, congress should remember this phrase: "Garbage in, garbage out."
- Looking at the list of celebrities that died over the past year, some deaths were related

to age and disease, some by accident, and some by substance abuse/overuse. The ones who died by substance abuse/overuse are just reminders for the rest of us, cautionary tales with no golden endings.

- Remember tonight is the night all the amateurs come out to party. Be safe and do not drink and drive.

- Lastly, another year passes and we remember those lost to us. I will raise a toast to Jody "Joe" Mateka, gone now twenty-six years as of this night and Jaymz Leland Hoburg gone now twenty-one years, among the many who have now passed.

To all the right wing zealots who claim the US was founded as a Christian nation by religious, church-going men...

Please say hello to a few of the Founding Fathers.

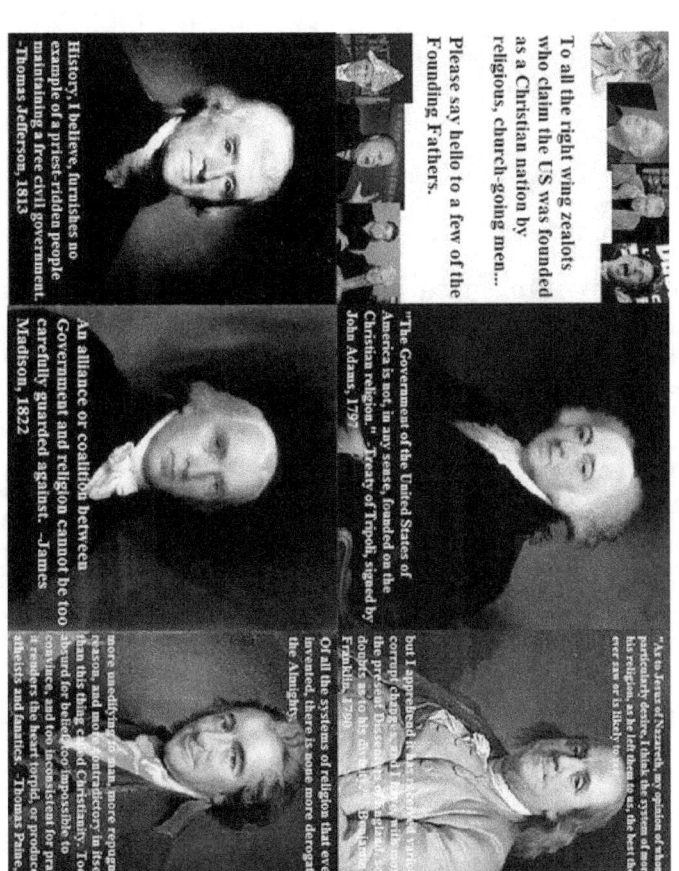

History, I believe, furnishes no example of a priest-ridden people maintaining a free civil government.
-Thomas Jefferson, 1813

"The Government of the United States of America is not, in any sense, founded on the Christian religion." -Treaty of Tripoli, signed by John Adams, 1797

An alliance or coalition between Government and religion cannot be too carefully guarded against. -James Madison, 1822

"As to Jesus of Nazareth, my opinion of whom you particularly desire, I think the system of morals and his religion, as he left them to us, the best the world ever saw or is likely to see..." -Benjamin Franklin, 1790

...but I apprehend it has received various corrupt changes, and I have, with most of the present Dissenters in England, some doubts as to his divinity...

Of all the systems of religion that ever were invented, there is none more derogatory to the Almighty, more unedifying to man, more repugnant to reason, and more contradictory in itself, than this thing called Christianity. Too absurd for belief, too impossible to convince, and too inconsistent for practice, it renders the heart torpid, or produces only atheists and fanatics. -Thomas Paine, 1795

21

Being a new dad once again

It is interesting being a new dad once again, considering my youngest is twenty years old now. First let me start by emphasizing that my fiancé and I were not expecting to have children, we thought we would grow old together as a pair of empty nesters, for doctors had told her that she would never successfully get pregnant, meaning carrying the fetus to term. She had had two miscarriages in her adult life, neither going past eight weeks of pregnancy. After the first sonogram, showing the fetus was attached to the uterus every day became a miracle. When we found out the baby's gender, our thoughts turned to giving it a name. Naming a child is not easy, you have to make sure of the spelling, how it will be pronounced, and its meaning and uniqueness. With each doctor's appointment, the upcoming birth of our child became closer to being a reality. My fiancé could not enjoy being pregnant due to the stress of gestational diabetes and a tightly controlled diet, being older meaning a high risk pregnancy, school (she is a nursing student), and the fact this was new territory for her. Each day, as I said earlier, became a minor miracle. Then at five months came the hard decisions if the genetic testing would show any abnormalities, we were lucky, no abnormalities, onward the pregnancy progressed.

Then at the thirty-nine week appointment, her blood pressure started to creep up, the doctor said within two days we would have a baby. We were told to check in to the hospital so the process could be started and within twenty-four hours we would have a newborn baby in our arms. Of course, the night we were to check in was a busy night in labor and delivery, after a nearly four-hour wait we were in a labor and delivery room and the birthing process begun. Everything was going well until the process stalled out when she was a nine centimeters, the baby had failed to enter the birth canal and a caesarian section was now necessary.

My thoughts drifted back to a day twenty-one years earlier when my first son was born and subsequently died due to a prolapsed umbilical cord (the cord was wrapped around his neck and strangled him, he was born brain dead and died within minutes) and the stress started to mount. I had to show a brave face and erase my fears to support my fiancé, to make sure she did not crack under the pressure. So far, the baby was fine and not in distress. Off she went to the operating room to be prepared for surgery and I was dressed in cap, gown, and booties to be by her side. With a screen to block of the view of her belly, and me sitting by her head listened to the doctor and assistant go through the process to remove the baby. Then we heard "we are removing the baby from the uterus," followed by a scream any heavy metal singer would be proud of, out came our son into the world. Over the screen the doctor flashed us our healthy child and the stress drained out of us, he made here and in good health.

Now the old and rusty skills were coming back, changing diapers, feeding, holding, burping, etc. and were being put to use. Right now, the biggest issue is getting on the baby's schedule as to feeding and sleeping but as a once again new parent I am up for the challenge; I am doing my part so my fiancé can continue her studies, and taking some of the stress off her. Every day is now an adventure, welcome my son, welcome to the machine.

How can we create change?

Change is terrifying. Change is necessary. Change can bring progress. Change does not lead to stagnation. Change can be easy. Change can be difficult. We can accept change or we can fight change but change is inevitable. You can be part of the solution and facilitate the change or you can be part of the problem and be why the change is happening. Change does not mean the end of things as we know them, change is the ushering in of a new era. Change can revitalize us or change can demoralize us only if we succumb to the despair that comes with loss. Change is a force for creativity, for forging a new tomorrow, and for enlightenment. Change is the only constant. Our universe is constantly changing. The seasons change. Change happens daily as darkness becomes light and as the daylight succumbs to the night. We can accept change or we can stagnate. Whichever path we choose we will change, the only question will be, "is the change of our own accord or are we being forced to change?"

What does the "Occupy Wall Street" movement want? What needs to change? How can we facilitate change? How can we make sure that the change benefits every one of us? How can we use change to prevent a repeat of what brought us to this point? What are the steps to the change? Will the change actually create change or will it just obfuscate the current situation. How can we lend our voices to the change?

I love my country but I dislike what those who hold the power do with that power and I fear that there is no difference between the two parties; the only difference is the packaging.

I do not begrudge those that achieve their success through hard work and perseverance. I do have an issue with those who achieve their success through smoke and mirrors or use the hard work of others to further their own ambitions and wealth.

Some insights into WHAT needs to change:

- Term limits on congress. I do not want to be president; I want to be a senator. The senate is where the real power in American politics is vested. To remove an incumbent senator is nearly impossible. No senator should serve long enough that two generations of voters have been born while they are in office. Our founding fathers envisioned a congress of public servants that would serve for a limited time then retire to their private life not individuals serving for the rest of their lives.

- Checks and balances put in place to prevent the financial collapse from repeating. We need to make sure that every citizen has faith in the financial industry. We need a strong financial industry to fuel the reawakening of American industry and the job market. We need the financial industry providing financing to small businesses, which are the backbone of American industry and provide the greatest number of jobs available in the workforce.

- We need congress voting their consciences and not along party lines. We need an end to partisan politics, our elected officials were elected to represent us, the voters and constituents, not pander to the elitist special interest groups backed by corporations. The difference between a politician and a patriot is a politician will do what will further their career and a patriot will do what is best for their country. As a country we need more patriots and fewer politicians, it is time for voters to quit being apathetic and express their opinions. Remember, if you do not exercise your right to vote then you have no right to complain about the job those elected are doing.

Randomness of thought...

Why is it when budget cuts come around education and educational programs are always on the chopping block? Is it any wonder why our children are failing behind the rest of the world? The United States used to be the pinnacle of education, now we are slowly sliding down the scale. Our funding of education needs to be a priority, fund the arts as well as the sciences, and quit pouring additional monies into sports programs. Path to education reform: Institute a uniform dress code, studies have found that public schools that have a "uniform" dress code have test scores rise over time, less instances of classroom disruptions, less instances of bullying, and students report less stress about going to school. Unfortunately, make interscholastic sports a "pay to play" system, if your student wants to play a particular sport you have to foot part of the bill. This is already happening around the country in smaller school districts that are strapped to fund regular classroom activities. Increase tax levies for education, educating the next generation should be priority number one not number one-thousand. Lastly, state academies for Math and Science, and for the Arts. Some areas and states already do this but every state needs to do this. Our education system is already one where the "haves" are getting more and the "haves not" are getting less; spending needs to equalize across the system.

Is sexting cheating? A better question is: Why would you want to send compromising pictures to someone else, who is not your partner, for the purpose of receiving similar pictures in return? In the internet age things can get spread rather quickly.

All religions attempt to explain our existence on this rock. Why should we argue over who is right when all boil down to "live a conscientious life" and "do no harm."

Your failure to act accordingly does not create an emergency for me or prompt me to take action.

If you sign up for something read the fine print, it is there for a reason.

Living healthy is expensive; no wonder we have become a nation of overweight couch potatoes.

Heard a commentator on the radio talking about if older generations had been "green" we would have less problems with the environment today. His comments did remind me of days gone by and how we were "green" then...I remember when beverages came in glass bottles and you returned those bottles for credit. I remember when the state of Iowa started giving $.05 cents refund on glass bottles and aluminum cans. You were also charged that refund amount extra at purchase. Doing a little research, in 1940, the average family produced about two tons of garbage per year, in 2000; the average family produced about ten tons of garbage per year. I remember when groceries left the store in paper bags, and those bags were the basis for art projects amongst other things. We walked or rode our bikes to school, the grocery store, to our friend's house, and not had mom drive us. I remember our garden, which provided fresh vegetables for the summer; and the canning and pickling of said vegetables in the fall; along with homemade grape jelly from our grape arbor. Learning to cook, pre-made and prepackaged foods were expensive and rather bland tasting. I used to think TV dinners (good ole Swansons meals in a tin tray) were an inducement for being well behaved for the sitter. Water came from the faucet or a fountain not a plastic bottle with some exotic name on it for a price.

What is wrong with this picture: 187 Teachers, Principles and other school administrators in the Atlanta, GA public school system are under investigation for manipulating standardized test results to show the school was helping the students improve as shown by the raising of test scores. Here is a symptom of a larger issue when it comes to handing out money to schools for the "increases" in test results, why would a school district need to do this? Simple answer: Our education system is floundering and needs to be overhauled in such a manner that our standards match the expectations. Think of these two facts: 1. Japan graduates more engineering students from their universities than any other nation. 2. The United States graduates more lawyers than all the European Union combined (roughly the same population).

Heard a discussion on the new law in Illinois on Civil Unions. Kudos to Illinois for tackling the issue of gay marriage in the right sense. The Civil Union is no different from a marriage both individuals have the same rights and protections under the law as any heterosexual couple has and by that standard, the marriage certificates in Illinois starting in 2012 will all be called Civil Union certificates. The State has separated marriage from civil union by using the language "the state has a right to grant the formation of a legal union between two consenting adults" and hands the matter of a marriage back to where it belongs, religious organizations. Marriage is a religious matter while the legal formation of a union is matter for the state, separate and different, one is for legal issues, and one is to satisfy one's religious beliefs.

Surfing again through the radio channels came across a discussion on the beginnings of the push to repeal the anti-polygamy laws in the U.S., which were created to specifically target the Mormon movement and part of the government agreement, which allowed Utah to become a state. Oddly enough the U.S. is one of the few G20 nations that have anti-polygamy laws, most countries do not specifically address it as a crime but place limits on the number of adult relationships within the family unit. Remembering what a Political Science professor had once said that the laws in the U.S. had their roots in the Puritan social beliefs and our national views were shaped by as such the religious right of center view on life in general. Work hard (nothing wrong with that), family first (nothing wrong again) and place god above all else and god's law (I do have a problem with this. Which god?) were the basic puritan tenets. Personally, I do not have a problem with polygamy or polyandry (wife with multiple husbands) as long as all parties involved are consenting adults and agree to the situation. It becomes a problem when one of the parties is neither consenting nor in agreement and is forced/coerced into the situation at hand. There is a movement called "polyamorous" which is very similar to polygamy but where two individuals have a legal marriage and the third (or extra partners) is a willing/consenting participant. The home situation is very similar to a polygamist household, shared family/household responsibilities and separate sexual relations among the adult members. This skirts the legal ramifications, meaning illegal polygamist activities, by not referencing the tertiary relationship as husband/wife but as partners, and all children of the household are taken care of and treated with equality. In some way as a nation, we need to look in the mirror and see if we like the face staring back at us. In our national discourse, we talk about freedoms but do we really want to grant them? As in the phrase "Life, liberty and the pursuit of happiness," are we willing to grant fringe groups equal rights or are we just blowing smoke?

Now with college football back in full swing it is time to take a swipe at the failed BCS championship format of D1-A schools. Here is an alternative (and please read all the way through before forming and opinion): An eleven-team playoff system. Why eleven teams? There are eleven D1-A football conferences and in this system only conference champions (as determined by each conference through championship game or round robin play) would qualify, all independent teams would not qualify no matter how good their record is (Sorry Notre Dame you need to join the Big East for all sports not for all sports but football) and which university they are. Here is how the playoff would go: First round six teams would play, eliminating three, after which there would eight teams left. Next rounds would go as follows round of eight (quarterfinals), round of four (semifinals), championship game. A total of ten games to be televised (imagine the dollars the NCAA would generate for this system) and would add a maximum of four games to any college teams' schedule. Rules to add/change: limit teams to eleven game seasons plus conference championship game, eliminate games between D1-A (FBS) schools and D1-AA (FCS) schools, and eliminate automatic bowl bids (set bowl eligibility at minimum of eight wins). With 33 bowl games each year, use some of the lower tier bowls as neutral sites for the first two rounds, and allow the conference runner-ups to go to the traditional bowl match ups. How would the teams be placed in the bracket? Prior to the start of the college football season a lottery would determine the placement of each conference on the championship bracket (eleven balls in a lottery machine randomly drawn one at a time then placed in one of the starting eleven spots). After all conference champions have been determined, the teams are plugged into the brackets based on their conference and play begins with one round of play each week for a total of four weeks of play. Why not expand this to sixteen teams? Simply too much controversy on who was added and who was left out, conference champions only get to play for a chance at a national title. This eliminates the controversy of power conferences (Big 10, Pac 10, Big 12, etc.) getting the spotlight versus the mid majors (MAC, Mountain West, Conference USA, etc.) best being jilted at bowl time. It is time for a true national championship game not a contrived convenience created by the BCS. As certain non-power conference schools have proved year after year they can play with anybody and beat them. You would think by now the NCAA has learned their lesson with all the revenue created by the NCAA Basketball tourney and apply that logic to football. D1-A football is the only major sport national title not determined by a playoff or sport appropriate system. It is time to get it correct NCAA, not time to create more controversy.

A great source of irony as our Soldiers, Sailors, Airmen, and Marines fight for the freedom of others along with our own freedoms, one of the freedoms upheld this year by the Supreme Court was the first Amendment. The Westboro Baptist Church that protests at the funerals of service personnel killed in combat or die as a result of said combat are allowed to protest at those funerals. Even though the spirit of the Amendment is being abused, the letter of the law is not; sad but true.

The Fractured Fairy Tale-The American Dream

I was born in the 1960's into a working middle class family.

I was raised in the 1970's by a stay at home mom and a father who was home after work, who was involved in my life.

- I grew up in a small town in western Illinois; a farming community, were hard work was prized. Success came by your own two hands, not on the back of someone else's labor and definitely not handed to you.

- Your neighbors helped your parents keep an eye on you and if you found trouble, there was no denying your part in it.

- Scouts, church, and the school were the guides to an upright and ethical life.

- Manners were expected and not to be forgotten. Common courtesy meant something, not to be practiced only when you felt like it but practiced all the time.

- When there was a difficult time, a death in the household or other tragedy, your neighbors helped, they were not afraid to lend a hand, or bring over food to feed you and yours.

I came of age in the 1980's, into a time when the selflessness of a generation, the baby boomers, brought greed and excess to the forefront.

- The rise of two income families and the coining of the term "latch key kids."

- The beginning of the breakdown of the idea of community, the beginning of when the phrase "fences make good neighbors."

- The beginning of the decline of our civilization, where manners and common courtesies were only reserved for friends and family and not extended to strangers, no way, no how, never to anyone you did not know.

- The rise of the Yuppie, where in the elitist neighborhood you had to keep pace with your neighbors and failure to do so was an unconscionable act. The rise of Suburbatory, cookie cutter houses, cookie cutter people with cookie cutter cubical jobs. Entire suburban areas that are essentially a boring bologna, processed cheese, and mayo sandwiches on white bread served with a side of blandness.

- In this time, I went away to college for the first time. Interesting enough it would have cost less for me to attend the University of Iowa instead of the University of Illinois, a two thousand dollar difference even paying out of state tuition. I did not choose either but a smaller in state public university at about one-sixth the cost of the University of Illinois.

I became a parent in the 1990's.

- Under educated and working with the skills I had acquired I was barely able to provide the necessities.

- In the decade of the 1990's we saw the rise of being "politically correct." The sanitizing of our society where speaking out and calling something what it was; for example, a lazy, unmotivated, and unemployed individual is not "economically challenged" and does not deserve to be coddled by society.

- We began to see the second and sometimes the third generation of welfare recipients continuing to perpetuate the "helplessness" and abuse the system.

- We see the gap begin to widen between those who have the wealth and those who are the working poor, the slow eroding of the middle class, and the booming cost of higher education.

At the turn of the twenty-first century, I was back in school, completing my education.

- I was beginning to see the light at the end of the tunnel. I was beginning to live the American dream of job security, family, middle class life style, and financial security.

- This was the decade of the eroding of our freedoms. An act of terror frightened us to the point that our government in the excuse of protecting us from outside threats began to attack our civil liberties.

- We, as a nation, became embroiled in wars in two sovereign nations with no clear options for victory or for withdrawal.

- I salute every soldier, sailor, marine, airman, and private citizen who has given all of themselves so others may be free of tyranny and so we, the common citizen, can go to sleep every night without fear and know someone out there is giving their all for our safety. We, as a nation, must honor these men and women when they return to our shores and we cannot forget those who returned in caskets or not at all.

- As the decade ended, we saw the collapse of our economy, a collapse fuel by greed and excess.

Now as the decade turns again we are in the midst of an economic downturn.

- The problem in a nutshell is this: Inequality in this country has hit a level that has been seen only once in the nation's history and unemployment has reached a level that has been seen only once since the Great Depression, and at the same time, corporate profits are at a record high. In other words, in the never-ending tug-of-war between "labor" and "capital," there has rarely, if ever, been a time when "capital" was so clearly winning.

- Citizens are protesting in the streets across our nation.

- If America cannot figure out a way to address the issues, the country will likely become increasingly "destabilized," as sociologists might say, and in that scenario, the current protests will likely be only the beginning.

- Let us start with the obvious: Unemployment. Three years after the financial crisis, the unemployment rate is still at the highest level since the Great Depression (except for a brief blip in the early 1980s).

- It is not that unemployment these days is a quick, painful jolt, a record percentage of unemployed people have been unemployed for longer than 6 months. It is not just construction workers who cannot find jobs, the median duration of all unemployment is also near an all-time high.

- Corporate profits as a percent of the economy are near a record all-time high. With the exception of a brief happy period in 2007 (just before the crash), profits are higher than they have been since the 1950s. They are vastly higher than they have been for most of the intervening half-century.

- The average CEO pay is now 350X the average worker's, up from 50X from 1960-1985.

- CEO pay has skyrocketed 300% since 1990. Corporate profits have doubled. Average "production worker" pay has increased 4%.

- While CEOs and shareholders have been cashing in, wages as a percent of the economy have dropped to an all-time low.

- Of course, life is great if you are in the top 1% of American wage earners. You are hauling in a bigger percentage of the country's total pre-tax income than you have at any time since the late 1920s. Your share of the national income, in fact, is almost two times the long-term average. In fact, income inequality has gotten so extreme here that the US now ranks 93rd (this is not a good metric by comparison Sweden's top 1% earns 23 times the income of an average worker while in US the top 1% on average earn 45 times the income of an average worker) in the world in "income equality." China is ahead of us. So is India. So is Iran.

- By the way, few people would have a problem with inequality if the American Dream were still intact, if it were easy to work your way into that top 1%. However, unfortunately, social mobility in this country is also near an all-time low.

- So what does all this mean in terms of net worth? Well, for starters, it means that the top 1% of Americans own 42% of the financial wealth in this country. The top 5%, meanwhile, own nearly 70%.

- HENRY's (High Earners, Not Rich Yet), most of whom are doctors, lawyers, and other professionals with loads of education related debt are suffering along with the average laborer. Think of this, nearly seventy-five percent of the work force earns below $50,000 a year.

- Remember that huge debt problem we have, with hundreds of millions of Americans indebted up to their eyeballs? Well, the top 1% does not have that problem; they only own 5% of the country's debt.

As I am a parent of grown children, a grandparent, and once again a parent to be, I fear that the American Dream will be no more than a fairy tale for the next generation with the exception of the top tier of society. The American dream will be for most only seen in the movies or on television, for the 99% of us we will become much like Robert DeNiro's character in *THX 182*, a parody of modern man.

We are nearing the tipping point of a crisis, a civil war between ideologies, between those who hold the wealth and political power and those struggling to make ends meet, between worker and corporation, between the government and the people. I do not advocate armed conflict; frankly, I would like to see it avoided. I would like to see change come through open dialogue and compromise between all parties involved but the pessimist in me thinks that will not happen without some physical conflict along the way. The optimist in me hopes we as a nation can come to an understanding and right our ship. The realist in me knows neither may happen or both may come to fruition, but either way we as a nation are in for a long and possibly rocky road ahead.

The Fractured Fairy Tale-The American Dream

I was born in the 1960's into a working middle class family.

I was raised in the 1970's by a stay at home mom and a father who was home after work, who was involved in my life.

- I grew up in a small town in western Illinois; a farming community, were hard work was prized. Success came by your own two hands, not on the back of someone else's labor and definitely not handed to you.

- Your neighbors helped your parents keep an eye on you and if you found trouble, there was no denying your part in it.

- Scouts, church, and the school were the guides to an upright and ethical life.

- Manners were expected and not to be forgotten. Common courtesy meant something, not to be practiced only when you felt like it but practiced all the time.

- When there was a difficult time, a death in the household or other tragedy, your neighbors helped, they were not afraid to lend a hand, or bring over food to feed you and yours.

I came of age in the 1980's, into a time when the selflessness of a generation, the baby boomers, brought greed and excess to the forefront.

- The rise of two income families and the coining of the term "latch key kids."

- The beginning of the breakdown of the idea of community, the beginning of when the phrase "fences make good neighbors."

- The beginning of the decline of our civilization, where manners and common courtesies were only reserved for friends and family and not extended to strangers, no way, no how, never to anyone you did not know.

- The rise of the Yuppie, where in the elitist neighborhood you had to keep pace with your neighbors and failure to do so was an unconscionable act. The rise of Suburbatory, cookie cutter houses, cookie cutter people with cookie cutter cubical jobs. Entire suburban areas that are essentially a boring bologna, processed cheese, and mayo sandwiches on white bread served with a side blandness.

- In this time, I went away to college for the first time. Interesting enough it would have cost less for me to attend the University of Iowa instead of the University of Illinois, a two thousand dollar difference even paying out of state tuition. I did not choose either but a smaller in state public university at about one-sixth the cost of the University of Illinois.

I became a parent in the 1990's.

- Under educated and working with the skills I had acquired I was barely able to provide the necessities.
- In the decade of the 1990's we saw the rise of being "politically correct." The sanitizing of our society where speaking out and calling something what it was; for example, a lazy, unmotivated, and unemployed individual is

not "economically challenged" and does not deserve to be coddled by society.

- We began to see the second and sometimes the third generation of welfare recipients continuing to perpetuate the "helplessness" and abuse the system.
- We see the gap begin to widen between those who have the wealth and those who are the working poor, the slow eroding of the middle class, and the booming cost of higher education.

At the turn of the twenty-first century, I was back in school, completing my education.

- I was beginning to see the light at the end of the tunnel. I was beginning to live the American dream of job security, family, middle class life style, and financial security.
- This was the decade of the eroding of our freedoms. An act of terror frightened us to the point that our government in the excuse of protecting us from outside threats began to attack our civil liberties.

- We, as a nation, became embroiled in wars in two sovereign nations with no clear options for victory or for withdrawal.
- I salute every soldier, sailor, marine, airman, and private citizen who has given all of themselves so others may be free of tyranny and so we, the common citizen, can go to sleep every night without fear and know someone out there is giving their all for our safety. We, as a nation, must honor these men and women when they return to our shores and we cannot forget those who returned in caskets or not at all.
- As the decade ended, we saw the collapse of our economy, a collapse fuel by greed and excess.

Now as the decade turns again we are in the midst of an economic downturn.

- The problem in a nutshell is this: Inequality in this country has hit a level that has been seen only once in the nation's history and unemployment has reached a level that has been seen only once since the Great Depression, and at the same time, corporate profits are at a record high. In other words, in the never-ending tug-of-war between "labor" and "capital," there has rarely, if ever, been a time when "capital" was so clearly winning.

- Citizens are protesting in the streets across our nation.

- If America cannot figure out a way to address the issues, the country will likely become increasingly "destabilized," as sociologists might say, and in that scenario, the current protests will likely be only the beginning.

- Let us start with the obvious: Unemployment. Three years after the financial crisis, the unemployment rate is still at the highest level since the Great Depression (except for a brief blip in the early 1980s).

- It is not that unemployment these days is a quick, painful jolt, a record percentage of unemployed people have been unemployed for longer than 6 months. It is not just construction workers who cannot find jobs, the median duration of all unemployment is also near an all-time high.

- Corporate profits as a percent of the economy are near a record all-time high. With the exception of a brief happy period in 2007 (just before the crash), profits are higher than they have been since the 1950s. They are vastly higher than they have been for most of the intervening half-century.

- The average CEO pay is now 350X the average worker's, up from 50X from 1960-1985.

- CEO pay has skyrocketed 300% since 1990. Corporate profits have doubled. Average "production worker" pay has increased 4%.

- While CEOs and shareholders have been cashing in, wages as a percent of the economy have dropped to an all-time low.

- Of course, life is great if you are in the top 1% of American wage earners. You are hauling in a bigger percentage of the country's total pre-tax income than you have at any time since the late 1920s. Your share of the national income, in fact, is almost two times the long-term average. In fact, income inequality has gotten so extreme here that the US now ranks 93rd (this is not a good metric by comparison Sweden's top 1% earns 23 times the income of an average worker while in US the top 1% on average earn 45 times the income of an average worker) in the world in "income equality." China is ahead of us. So is India. So is Iran.

- By the way, few people would have a problem with inequality if the American Dream were still intact, if it were easy to work your way into that top 1%. However, unfortunately, social mobility in this country is also near an all-time low.

- So what does all this mean in terms of net worth? Well, for starters, it means that the top 1% of Americans own 42% of the financial wealth in this country. The top 5%, meanwhile, own nearly 70%.

- HENRY's (High Earners, Not Rich Yet), most of whom are doctors, lawyers, and other professionals with loads of education related debt are suffering along with the average laborer. Think of this, nearly seventy-five percent of the work force earns below $50,000 a year.

- Remember that huge debt problem we have, with hundreds of millions of Americans indebted up to their eyeballs? Well, the top 1% does not have that problem; they only own 5% of the country's debt.

As I am a parent of grown children, a grandparent, and once again a parent to be, I fear that the American Dream will be no more than a fairy tale for the next generation with the exception of the top tier of society. The American dream will be for most only seen in the movies or on television, for the 99% of us we will become much like Robert DeNiro's character in *THX 182*, a parody of modern man.

We are nearing the tipping point of a crisis, a civil war between ideologies, between those who hold the wealth and political power and those struggling to make ends meet, between worker and corporation, between the government and the people. I do not advocate armed conflict; frankly, I would like to see it avoided. I would like to see change come through open dialogue and compromise between all parties involved but the pessimist in me thinks that will not happen without some physical conflict along the way. The optimist in me hopes we as a nation can come to an understanding and right our ship. The realist in me knows neither may happen or both may come to fruition, but either way we as a nation are in for a long and possibly rocky road ahead.

Where does gravity fall?

A collection of poetry that I have written over the years for your enjoyment, sit back and read.

This first piece I wrote during my freshman year of college while taking a creative writing class. It is a tribute to friend of mine who died New Years eve, six months after we had graduated high school.

Snowflakes

Why do they come?

Drifting, falling in downward flight,

To some they are welcome,

As they fall to earth tonight.

The whiteness has turned to grey,

The sky was blue,

"What might he say?"

Someone would ask you.

And now all is dark,

"For was it right?"

I have heard the meadowlark

Cry out it the night.

"Was it his time to die?

And soon shall I?"

Life goes on through the days,

He no longer walks by my side,

As we wander through the fields of hay.

This brother of mine took a ride,

To the worlds above the ground.

In the time of night,

One might look around,

And see that he was right.

Peace be with you,

Brother of mine,

You venture to a world of new,

Where you will remember the time of nine.

"Weep not for me,"

Says he, "Remember what it is to be."

Another poem from that same time...

Self Portrait #1

Only the looking glass can show the three,
Me, myself, and I.

Stone cold he is,
Diabolical in every way.
Savage and lustful,
Cold and calculating,
The mind is his realm.

Only his reality is true,
Pain and comfort control him.
His doings are the effects of the others.
He knows no love nor hatred,
Only the consequences,
The body is his realm.

Gentle he is,
Chivalry is his code,
Love and caring are his actions.
He is spiritual,
Seeking out knowledge and truth,

The soul is his realm.

These three,
Me, myself, and I,
Are the body, mind, and soul.
None can live without the others,
All are strong,
And yet all are weak.

The mind and soul struggle,
To control the body,
And it seems,
One shall become strong,
While the other is weak.
And so on the two battle...

Look into the mirror and see
Which is strong and which is weak.

The following is a collection of untitled works that I have written over the last twenty-five or so years.

Untitled #1

When the moon breaks the horizon,

When the night begins to gather,

You'll find us there,

At the edge of your vision,

Sliding in and out of the shadows.

Wolf brothers we are

And will be,

The guardians of the night,

The protectors of the innocents,

The watchers,

The warriors,

The pack.

Untitled #2

Minstrel of fate play a new song for me,

I have heard your songs all my life,

And yet they seem ever new.

I pray for a sad song,

A song of sorrow,

One of sickness,

Of pestilence, of death.

For I cannot explain these feelings,

Inside of me,

The pain and distrust.

I hurt not for myself

But for others in this world

Whom are without family, food or home.

The ones who daily call out to you

For the song of mourning and death.

Hear me O minstrel let all who sit in this land

At one time or another with a gluttonous, hedonistic,

pish posh view,

Feel the pain of the others.

Play your song of harmony, balance, and peace…

Untitled #3

What do you do when you think

The whole world is laughing at you?

Do you cry?

Or take a walk and wonder why?

Am I small and insignificant?

No!

Can I fly above

And conquer them all?

Yes!

The sounds of the world

Form music in my mind,

A melody that I pull from the air,

That makes me strong with time.

Just being alone in the crowd

With a song in your mind

That you sing to yourself

Is just being alone in the crowd

And nothing is wrong.

Untitled #4

Life,

A two bit whore in heat,

Always looking for some john

Who will give her more than she deserves.

Five, ten, and if she's lucky maybe a twenty.

But all she wants

Is a piece of action

Your body,

Your life.

Full of disease and death.

Untitled #5

Hear the snow

Watching it drift down

From the sky

Piling up

Around my feet

Deep it is

Cleansing me

And the world too

Good it is

This is the poem that will one day become a song of mine by the same title.

Travelling man

It seems like I have been here before

But I don't know why

For every town on the road looks the same

Only the faces

Faces seem to change

But I think I've been here before

But I don't know why

Last night I was in this town along the road

All the faces seem familiar

But I don't know why

There was a girl

Whom seemed to know me

But they always do

Maybe I've been here before

But I don't know why

For every town on the road looks the same

The road has been so long

Every inn seems like home

Maybe someday I'll be caught by a travelling woman

Then the road won't seem so long anymore

Maybe we will wattle down

And start a family

But right now I am still rolling down the road

The road has been to long

And it is wearing me down

I am going to lie down

And get some sleep maybe when I wake up

I will be in the next town again.

Infinite Odyssey

We had nothing to do but start a time,

A time with a beginning

And yet without an end,

But yet it had an end,

Without a beginning.

It was our odyssey

Without any dimension.

It was a time

When world were created

And those that existed were destroyed

See that star the one flickering red

Tomorrow it will be gone in a flash

Here we are travelling like Ulysses

On an odyssey in space

Could it be that we will not see home again

In twenty millennia

Can you hear her?

The siren of space

She is luring you to an airless grave

That no one will find until the end of time.

It is only a dream

Space is not real

It is just call of ages old

To search the heavens

In our time of discovery

The power of time will be lost

To those who are unready

We shall lead the way

On this space odyssey

The time

The dimension

The end of the worlds

Pilot

Lead the way the in forgotten time

Since time no longer exist

We need not worry about being late

Since supper will not be ready

Lead us to the end for there was no beginning.

Which way for a Witch?

Which way for a witch?

Boil, boil, toil, and trouble,

Is it double?

Dancing in the moonlight?

Or sunshine in the glade?

Carousing at a faire,

Or fairly carousing?

Turn a charm,

Or taking a charming turn?

Life's questions must be met,

Head on in this unwitchy world.

For solitary selves we must be,

To survive amongst the flock.

Eagles in a world of ducks

Soaring above constraints

Of ignorance and injustice.

So?

Which way for a witch?

This last piece was another ode to a friend who died.

Death of a friend

She was more loyal to me

Than most women in my life

I saved her once from death

But was powerless this time

In the end it was right, euthanasia

For my friend

She need not suffer anymore

For she had done enough

Good bye my friend

And remember not to pee on the tree of life

My most loyal four legged friend,
Maxine.

OWS Protest Beans

Ingredients:

- (2) 16oz cans of black beans or white navy beans, drained and rinsed
- 4 cups of water
- 1 tablespoon of minced garlic
- 2 jalapeno peppers, seeded and minced
- 1 teaspoon of salt
- 1 teaspoon of ground black pepper
- 1 teaspoon of dried cilantro
- 1 tablespoon of olive oil
- 2 cups of long grain rice
- (1) 8oz can of tomato sauce
- (1) 16oz can of diced tomatoes
- 1 teaspoon of onion powder

In a Crockpot set on high or stockpot with a lid:

1. Place olive oil and garlic in pot and cook until garlic starts to turn brown.
2. Add all other ingredients except the rice to the pot.
3. Bring to a boil then reduce heat to a simmer, and cover.

4. Cook for 1 hour.
5. Add rice and continue to cook until rice is tender, about 20 minutes.
6. Serve hot with cornbread or crusty bread.

I cannot always be down at the OWS protest but I can help, and do my part by providing a warm meal to those who are spending all their time there.

- I am of the 99%.
- Do not call me a hippy or lazy because I am unemployed.
- I have a Masters degree in business but you of the 1% tell me that I should be thankful for a minimum wage job. Net monthly income on minimum wage (if you work 40 hours per week) is approximately $936 after taxes and before any benefits (if offered) are subtracted.
- Average debt carried by college graduates is twenty-five thousand of college related

expense, estimated time to pay off these expenses is a minimum of fifteen years.

- About 70% of high school students go on for further education but only about 25% graduate with a bachelors degree. For easy numbers approximately 18 students out of every 100 students who graduate high school also earn a bachelors degree from a college or university.

- Think about this: Nationally 82% of the US workforce is uneducated or undereducated. Approximately 47% of US workers earn under $25k/year and approximately 75% of US workers earn under $50k/year and approximately 6% of US workers earn over $100k/year; average household expenses for a family of four equates to 77% of gross income and average family income is approximately $62k/year so expenses equate to $48k/year.